CIRRHOSIS COOKBOOK FOR NEWLY DIAGNOSED

Easy-to-Make and Nutritious Meal Plans to Manage Symptoms and Improve Liver Health

Sonia Emmason

CHAPTER 1

Cirrhosis is a condition in which the liver becomes damaged and scarred over time. This can happen due to a variety of causes, including chronic alcohol abuse, hepatitis, fatty liver disease, or autoimmune diseases. When the liver is damaged, it becomes less able to perform its crucial functions, such as filtering toxins from the blood, producing bile to help with digestion, and regulating blood sugar levels. As a result, individuals with cirrhosis may experience a range of symptoms, including fatigue, weakness, nausea, vomiting, jaundice, and swelling in the abdomen and legs.

While there is no cure for cirrhosis, there are steps that individuals can take to manage their symptoms and slow the progression of the disease. One of the most important aspects of managing cirrhosis is following a healthy diet that supports liver function and reduces the workload on the liver.

This Cirrhosis Diet for Newly Diagnosed is designed to provide nutritional guidance and delicious recipes for individuals who have been recently diagnosed with cirrhosis. This cookbook includes information on the types of foods that are beneficial for liver health, as well as those that should be avoided or limited.

The main goals of this Cirrhosis Diet for Newly Diagnosed are to:

1. **Provide essential nutrients:** The liver requires a variety of vitamins and minerals to function properly. These include vitamins A, D, E, K, and B-complex vitamins, as well as minerals like iron, zinc, and magnesium. The cookbook includes recipes that are rich in these nutrients, such as leafy greens, whole grains, lean protein, and healthy fats.

2. **Reduce inflammation:** Inflammation is a major contributor to liver damage in cirrhosis. Certain foods, such as processed foods, sugar, and alcohol, can increase inflammation in the body. The cookbook focuses on anti-inflammatory foods,

such as fruits, vegetables, nuts, and seeds, that can help reduce inflammation and support liver health.

3. **Manage symptoms:** Individuals with cirrhosis may experience a range of symptoms, such as nausea, vomiting, and bloating. The cookbook includes recipes that are easy to digest and can help manage these symptoms, such as soups, smoothies, and small, frequent meals.

4. **Support weight management:** Maintaining a healthy weight is important for individuals with cirrhosis, as excess weight can increase the workload on the liver. The cookbook includes recipes that are nutrient-dense but low in calories, such as salads, grilled vegetables, and lean protein.

In addition to providing delicious recipes, this Cirrhosis Diet for Newly Diagnosed also includes tips for meal planning, grocery shopping, and food preparation. It also provides information on how to read nutrition labels and make healthy choices when eating out.

While following a healthy diet is an important aspect of managing cirrhosis, it is also important to work closely with a healthcare provider to develop a comprehensive treatment plan. This may include medications, lifestyle changes, and monitoring for complications such as liver cancer or liver failure.

Overall, this Cirrhosis Diet for Newly Diagnosed is a valuable resource for individuals with cirrhosis who are looking to improve their liver health and manage their symptoms. By following the nutritional guidance and recipes in this cookbook, individuals can take an active role in their health and well-being.

CHAPTER 2

2.0 UNDERSTANDING CIRRHOSIS

2.1 WHAT IS CIRRHOSIS?

Cirrhosis is a condition in which the liver becomes scarred and damaged over time, leading to a decline in its ability to function properly. The liver is a vital organ that performs a number of crucial functions, including filtering toxins from the blood, producing bile to help with digestion, and regulating blood sugar levels. When the liver becomes damaged and scarred, it is less able to perform these functions, which can lead to a variety of symptoms and complications.

Cirrhosis can be caused by a number of factors, including chronic alcohol abuse, viral hepatitis, fatty liver disease, autoimmune diseases, and certain genetic disorders. In some cases, the cause of cirrhosis may be unknown.

The progression of cirrhosis varies from person to person and depends on the underlying cause of the disease.

In some cases, cirrhosis may progress slowly over many years, while in others it may progress more rapidly. As cirrhosis progresses, individuals may experience symptoms such as fatigue, weakness, nausea, vomiting, jaundice (yellowing of the skin and eyes), and swelling in the abdomen and legs.

In addition to these symptoms, cirrhosis can also lead to complications such as portal hypertension (high blood pressure in the veins that carry blood to the liver), esophageal varices (enlarged veins in the esophagus), hepatic encephalopathy (a build-up of toxins in the brain), and liver cancer.

Treatment for cirrhosis depends on the underlying cause of the disease and the severity of the damage to the liver. In some cases, lifestyle changes such as quitting alcohol or losing weight may be recommended. Medications may also be prescribed to manage symptoms or to slow the progression of the disease. In severe cases, a liver transplant may be necessary.

Cirrhosis is a condition in which the liver becomes damaged and scarred over time, leading to a decline in its ability to function properly. There are a variety of factors that can contribute to the development of cirrhosis, including:

1. **Chronic alcohol abuse**: Long-term alcohol consumption can lead to alcoholic liver disease, which can progress to cirrhosis over time.

2. **Viral hepatitis:** Hepatitis B and C are viral infections that can cause inflammation of the liver and, over time, lead to cirrhosis.

3. **Non-alcoholic fatty liver disease (NAFLD):** This condition occurs when there is a build-up of fat in the liver, often due to factors such as obesity, diabetes, or high cholesterol. In some cases, NAFLD can progress to cirrhosis.

4. **Autoimmune diseases:** Autoimmune diseases such as autoimmune hepatitis, primary biliary cholangitis, and primary sclerosing cholangitis

can cause inflammation and damage to the liver, which can lead to cirrhosis over time.

5. **Inherited liver diseases:** Certain genetic conditions, such as hemochromatosis (a condition that causes excess iron to build up in the liver) or Wilson's disease (a condition that causes excess copper to accumulate in the liver), can lead to cirrhosis over time.

6. **Chronic viral infections:** Chronic infections with viruses such as HIV or hepatitis D can also lead to cirrhosis.

7. **Biliary cirrhosis:** This type of cirrhosis occurs when there is damage to the bile ducts, which can lead to a buildup of bile in the liver and ultimately to cirrhosis.

It's worth noting that not everyone who has one of these risk factors will develop cirrhosis, and in many cases the development of cirrhosis may be influenced by other factors such as age, gender, overall health, and lifestyle factors such as diet and exercise.

If you suspect that you may be at risk for cirrhosis, it's important to speak with a healthcare provider to discuss screening and preventative measures.

Cirrhosis is a progressive liver disease that develops slowly over time. The symptoms of cirrhosis may not be noticeable in the early stages of the disease, and they can vary depending on the severity of the condition. Some common signs and symptoms of cirrhosis include:

1. **Fatigue and weakness:** As the liver becomes more damaged, it may become less effective at processing nutrients and producing energy, leading to feelings of fatigue and weakness.

2. **Jaundice:** A yellowing of the skin and whites of the eyes, known as jaundice, can occur when the liver is not functioning properly and bilirubin (a waste product) builds up in the blood.

3. **Abdominal swelling:** As cirrhosis progresses, it can lead to a buildup of fluid in the abdomen, a condition known as ascites. This can cause abdominal swelling and discomfort.

4. **Easy bruising and bleeding:** The liver produces clotting factors that help to prevent bleeding. When the liver is damaged, these clotting factors

may not be produced properly, leading to easy bruising and bleeding.

5. **Itchy skin:** In some cases, cirrhosis can cause itching due to a buildup of bile products in the blood.

6. **Changes in appetite and weight loss:** As cirrhosis progresses, it can lead to a loss of appetite and unintentional weight loss.

7. **Confusion and memory problems:** When the liver is not functioning properly, it can lead to a buildup of toxins in the blood that can affect brain function, leading to confusion, memory problems, and even coma in severe cases.

8. **Spider veins:** Cirrhosis can cause small, spider-like blood vessels to appear on the skin.

It's important to note that not everyone with cirrhosis will experience all of these symptoms, and some people may not experience any symptoms at all until the disease has progressed significantly. If you have any concerns about your liver health or are experiencing any of these symptoms, it's important to speak with a healthcare provider for an evaluation and appropriate treatment.

2.4 DIAGNOSIS OF CIRRHOSIS

Cirrhosis is a chronic liver disease that occurs when healthy liver tissue is replaced by scar tissue, leading to liver dysfunction. It can be diagnosed through a combination of medical history, physical examination, and laboratory tests.

Some common diagnostic tools and tests used to diagnose cirrhosis include:

1. **Medical history and physical examination:** A doctor will ask questions about the patient's medical history and symptoms and perform a physical exam to check for signs of liver damage, such as an enlarged liver or spleen, yellowing of the skin or eyes (jaundice), or spider-like blood vessels on the skin.

2. **Blood tests:** Blood tests can be used to check liver function and identify liver damage. These tests may include liver function tests, which measure

levels of liver enzymes, bilirubin, and other substances in the blood, as well as tests for hepatitis B and C viruses and other liver diseases.

3. **Imaging tests:** Imaging tests, such as ultrasound, CT scan, or MRI, can be used to examine the liver and detect signs of cirrhosis, such as nodules, scarring, or fluid buildup.

4. **Biopsy:** A liver biopsy involves removing a small sample of liver tissue for examination under a microscope. This test can help confirm a diagnosis of cirrhosis and identify the underlying cause.

It's important to note that cirrhosis can develop over time, and many people with the condition may not experience symptoms until the disease has progressed. As a result, regular screening and monitoring are important for people at risk of developing cirrhosis, such as those with chronic liver diseases, heavy alcohol use, or obesity.

2.5 COMPLICATIONS OF CIRRHOSIS

Cirrhosis is a serious and progressive condition that can lead to various complications, including:

1. **Portal hypertension:** Cirrhosis can cause high blood pressure in the portal vein, which carries blood from the digestive organs to the liver. This can lead to the development of varices, or enlarged veins, in the esophagus, stomach, or intestines, which can rupture and cause life-threatening bleeding.

2. **Ascites:** Cirrhosis can also cause fluid buildup in the abdomen, called ascites. This can cause abdominal swelling, discomfort, and difficulty breathing.

3. **Hepatic encephalopathy:** When the liver is damaged, it may not be able to remove toxins from the blood, which can lead to a buildup of these toxins in the brain, causing confusion, disorientation, and other neurological symptoms.

4. **Liver cancer:** People with cirrhosis are at increased risk of developing liver cancer.

5. **Malnutrition:** Cirrhosis can affect the liver's ability to store and process nutrients, leading to malnutrition and weight loss.

6. **Coagulation disorders:** The liver produces several proteins that are important for blood clotting. In cirrhosis, the liver may not produce enough of these proteins, leading to bleeding disorders.

7. **Increased risk of infections:** The liver plays a key role in fighting infections. In cirrhosis, the immune system may be weakened, leading to an increased risk of infections.

These complications can be serious and potentially life-threatening. People with cirrhosis should work closely with their healthcare provider to manage their condition and prevent complications.

CHAPTER 3

3.0 NUTRITION AND DIET FOR THE NEWLY DIAGNOSED

3.1 NUTRITION AND DIET GUIDELINES FOR CIRRHOSIS

Nutrition and diet play an important role in the management of cirrhosis. Here are some general guidelines:

1. **Limit sodium intake:** People with cirrhosis are at increased risk of developing ascites, a condition where fluid builds up in the abdomen. Reducing sodium intake can help prevent or manage ascites. The recommended daily sodium intake for people with cirrhosis is typically less than 2,000 mg.

2. **Eat a balanced diet:** A balanced diet that includes plenty of fruits, vegetables, whole grains, lean proteins, and healthy fats can help support liver function and overall health.

3. **Limit alcohol intake:** Alcohol can further damage the liver, so people with cirrhosis should avoid or limit alcohol consumption.

4. **Consider protein intake:** People with cirrhosis may be advised to limit protein intake if they have hepatic encephalopathy, a condition where the liver is unable to remove toxins from the blood. However, some protein is still necessary for maintaining muscle mass and supporting overall health, so protein intake should be managed on a case-by-case basis.

5. **Consider vitamin and mineral supplements:** Cirrhosis can affect the body's ability to absorb and store vitamins and minerals. People with cirrhosis may be advised to take supplements, such as vitamin D or calcium, to prevent deficiencies.

6. **Consult a registered dietitian:** A registered dietitian can help create an individualized nutrition plan that meets the specific needs and preferences of a person with cirrhosis.

For people with cirrhosis, it is important to avoid or limit certain foods and beverages that can be harmful to the liver and exacerbate the condition. Here are some foods and beverages to avoid or limit:

1. **Alcohol:** People with cirrhosis should avoid alcohol completely as it can further damage the liver.

2. **Sodium-rich foods:** High-sodium foods can cause fluid buildup in the body, worsening ascites and swelling. Foods to limit or avoid include canned soups, processed meats, pickles, salty snacks, and fast food.

3. **Fatty and fried foods:** These can be difficult for the liver to process and can contribute to liver damage. Foods to limit or avoid include fried foods, high-fat meats, full-fat dairy products, and fast food.

4. **Red meat:** High levels of protein and iron in red meat can put extra strain on the liver. It is recommended to limit red meat consumption and

choose leaner protein sources, such as fish, chicken, and plant-based proteins.

5. **Raw or undercooked shellfish:** Shellfish can contain bacteria and viruses that can be harmful to people with cirrhosis, who may have weakened immune systems. It is recommended to cook shellfish thoroughly to reduce the risk of infection.

6. **Grapefruit and grapefruit juice:** These can interfere with the liver's ability to metabolize certain medications, which can be especially problematic for people with cirrhosis who may be taking multiple medications.

7. **Sugary foods and beverages:** These can contribute to weight gain and fatty liver disease, which can worsen cirrhosis. Foods to limit or avoid include sugary drinks, desserts, and processed snacks.

It's important to note that the dietary needs and restrictions for people with cirrhosis can vary depending on the severity of the condition and the presence of complications.

3.3 FOODS TO ENJOY

For people with cirrhosis, it's important to focus on a well-balanced and nutritious diet. Here are some foods that can be included as part of a healthy diet:

Fruits and vegetables: These are important sources of vitamins, minerals, and fiber. Aim for a variety of colors and types, including leafy greens, berries, citrus fruits, and cruciferous vegetables like broccoli and cauliflower.

Whole grains: These are good sources of fiber, which can help support digestion and overall health. Choose whole-grain bread, pasta, and cereal.

Lean protein sources: These are important for building and repairing muscle and supporting overall health. Good sources include fish, chicken, turkey, tofu, and legumes like beans and lentils.

Low-fat dairy products: These can be a good source of calcium and other important nutrients. Choose low-fat or fat-free options, such as milk, yogurt, and cheese.

Healthy fats: These are important for overall health and can help support liver function.

Good sources include nuts, seeds, avocado, olive oil, and fatty fish like salmon and sardines.

Water: Staying hydrated is important for overall health and can help prevent fluid buildup in the body. Aim for at least 8-10 cups of water per day, or more if advised by a healthcare provider.

Herbal tea: Some herbal teas, such as green tea or chamomile tea, may have anti-inflammatory properties and may be beneficial for people with cirrhosis.

It's important to note that the dietary needs and recommendations for people with cirrhosis can vary depending on the severity of the condition and the presence of complications.

CHAPTER 4

Ingredients:

-1/2 cup rolled oats

-1 cup milk or non-dairy milk of choice

-1/4 teaspoon cinnamon

-1 tablespoon honey

-1/2 cup of fresh or frozen fruit (berries, banana, apples, etc.)

Instructions:

1. In a medium-sized pot, bring the milk to a boil over medium-high heat.

2. Stir in the oats and reduce the heat to low.

3. Simmer for 5 minutes, stirring occasionally.

4. Stir in the cinnamon and honey.

5. Add the fruit and cook for another 5 minutes.

6. Serve with a sprinkle of nuts or seeds for extra nutrition.

Ingredients:

-1 cup plain Greek yogurt

-1/4 cup nuts or seeds

-1/4 cup dried fruit

-1/4 cup fresh fruit

Instructions:

1. In a bowl, layer the yogurt, nuts/seeds, dried fruit and fresh fruit.

2. Serve chilled or at room temperature.

Ingredients:

-1 cup spinach

-1/2 cup almond milk

-1/2 avocado

-1/2 banana

-1 tablespoon honey

Instructions:

1. Place all ingredients in a blender and blend until smooth.

2. Serve chilled or at room temperature.

Ingredients:

-2 slices of whole wheat bread

-1 scrambled egg

-1 slice of cheese

Instructions:

1. Toast the bread in a toaster or in a pan over medium heat until lightly browned.

2. Meanwhile, scramble the egg in a pan over medium heat.

3. Place the scrambled egg and cheese on one slice of bread.

4. Top with the other slice of bread and serve.

Ingredients:

-1 whole wheat tortilla

-1/4 cup cooked black beans

-1/4 cup cooked brown rice

-1/4 cup diced bell pepper

-1 scrambled egg

Instructions:

1. Heat the tortilla in a pan over medium heat.

2. In a bowl, mix together the black beans, brown rice, bell pepper and egg.

3. Place the mixture in the center of the tortilla and fold the sides of the tortilla up to form a burrito.

4. Serve warm.

Ingredients:

-1 whole wheat tortilla

-1/4 cup cooked black beans

-1/4 cup cooked brown rice

-1/4 cup diced bell pepper

-1/4 cup shredded cheese

Instructions:

1. Heat the tortilla in a pan over medium heat.

2. In a bowl, mix together the black beans, brown rice, bell pepper and cheese.

3. Place the mixture in the center of the tortilla and fold the sides of the tortilla up to form a quesadilla.

4. Cook in the pan over medium heat until the cheese is melted and the quesadilla is lightly browned.

5. Serve warm.

Ingredients:

-1/2 cup rolled oats

-1/2 cup milk or non-dairy milk of choice

-1 tablespoon honey

-1/4 cup nuts or seeds

-1/4 cup dried fruit

Instructions:

1. Place the oats, milk and honey in a bowl and mix together.

2. Add the nuts/seeds and dried fruit and mix again.

3. Cover the bowl with plastic wrap and refrigerate overnight.

4. Serve chilled or at room temperature.

Ingredients:

-1 cup whole wheat flour

-1 teaspoon baking powder

-1/2 teaspoon baking soda

-1/4 teaspoon salt

-1 cup milk or non-dairy milk of choice

-2 tablespoons honey

-2 tablespoons vegetable oil

Instructions:

1. In a medium-sized bowl, mix together the flour, baking powder, baking soda and salt.

2. In a separate bowl, mix together the milk, honey and oil.

3. Pour the wet ingredients into the dry ingredients and mix until just combined.

4. Heat a non-stick pan over medium heat.

5. Pour 1/4 cup of the batter into the pan and cook until the edges are golden brown and the center is set.

6. Flip the pancake and cook until the other side is golden brown.

7. Serve hot with your favorite toppings.

Ingredients:

-2 eggs

-1/4 cup diced bell pepper

-1/4 cup diced onion

-1/4 cup diced mushrooms

-1 tablespoon olive oil

Instructions:

1. Heat the olive oil in a pan over medium heat.

2. Add the bell pepper, onion and mushrooms and cook for 3-4 minutes.

3. Crack the eggs into the pan and scramble with the vegetables until the eggs are cooked through.

4. Serve warm.

Ingredients:

-2 slices of whole wheat bread

-2 tablespoons nut butter (almond, cashew, peanut, etc.)

-1 banana, sliced

Instructions:

1. Toast the bread in a toaster or in a pan over medium heat until lightly browned.

2. Spread the nut butter over the toast.

3. Top with the banana slices.

4. Serve warm.

Ingredients:

- 4 ounces salmon fillet

- 2 tablespoons olive oil

- Salt and pepper to taste

- 2 cups baby spinach

- 1/2 cup cooked brown rice

- 2 tablespoons butter

- 1/4 cup chopped onion

- 1/4 cup chopped celery

- 1/4 cup chopped carrots

Instructions:

1. Preheat the grill to medium-high heat.

2. Brush the salmon with the olive oil and season with salt and pepper.

3. Grill the salmon for 4-5 minutes per side.

4. In a large skillet, heat the butter over medium-high heat.

5. Add the onion, celery, and carrots and cook for 3-4 minutes, stirring occasionally.

6. Add the spinach and cook until wilted, about 2 minutes.

7. Add the cooked brown rice and combine.

8. Serve the salmon with the sautéed spinach and brown rice pilaf.

9. Enjoy!

Ingredients:

- 1 whole wheat pita pocket

- 2 slices turkey breast

- 2 slices tomato

- 2 slices lettuce

- 2 tablespoons mayonnaise

- 2 tablespoons mustard

Instructions:

1. Slice the pita pocket open and spread the mayonnaise and mustard inside.

2. Place the turkey, tomato, and lettuce slices inside the pita pocket.

3. Close the pita pocket and cut in half.

4. Enjoy!

Ingredients:

- 1/2 cup cooked quinoa

- 1/4 cup diced cucumber

- 1/4 cup diced tomato

- 1/4 cup diced red onion

- 1/4 cup sliced black olives

- 2 tablespoons olive oil

- 2 tablespoons lemon juice

- Salt and pepper to taste

Instructions:

1. In a large bowl, combine the quinoa, cucumber, tomato, red onion, and black olives.

2. In a small bowl, whisk together the olive oil, lemon juice, salt, and pepper.

3. Pour the dressing over the quinoa mixture and toss to combine.

4. Serve the quinoa bowl.

5. Enjoy!

4. Veggie Stir-Fry (20 minutes)

Ingredients:

- 2 tablespoons olive oil

- 1 cup sliced mushrooms

- 1 cup sliced bell peppers

- 1 cup sliced carrots

- 1 cup sliced zucchini

- 1/4 cup soy sauce

- Salt and pepper to taste

Instructions:

1. Heat the olive oil in a large skillet over medium-high heat.

2. Add the mushrooms, bell peppers, carrots, and zucchini and cook until tender, about 5 minutes.

3. Add the soy sauce and season with salt and pepper.

4. Stir to combine and cook for an additional 2 minutes.

5. Serve the stir-fry.

6. Enjoy!

Ingredients:

- 2 cups cooked tortellini

- 1/3 cup sun-dried tomatoes

- 2 tablespoons olive oil

- 2 tablespoons balsamic vinegar

- 1/4 cup chopped basil

- Salt and pepper to taste

Instructions:

1. In a large bowl, combine the cooked tortellini, sun-dried tomatoes, olive oil, balsamic vinegar, and basil.

2. Season with salt and pepper.

3. Toss to combine.

4. Serve the tortellini salad.

5. Enjoy!

Ingredients:

- 2 slices whole wheat bread

- 1/2 avocado, mashed

- 2 hard-boiled eggs, sliced

- 1 cup baby spinach

- Salt and pepper to taste

Instructions:

1. Spread the mashed avocado on one slice of bread.

2. Top with the sliced eggs, spinach, and season with salt and pepper.

3. Top with the other slice of bread.

4. Cut in half and serve.

5. Enjoy!

Ingredients:

- 1 whole wheat wrap

- 2 tablespoons hummus

- 1/4 cup sliced cucumber

- 1/4 cup sliced bell peppers

- 1/4 cup sliced carrots

- 1/4 cup sliced radishes

- Salt and pepper to taste

Instructions:

1. Spread the hummus on the wrap.

2. Top with the cucumber, bell peppers, carrots, and radishes.

3. Season with salt and pepper.

4. Roll the wrap up and cut in half.

5. Serve the wrap.

6. Enjoy!

Ingredients:

- 1 can tuna, drained

- 1/4 cup sliced green beans

- 1/4 cup sliced tomatoes

- 1/4 cup sliced red onion

- 2 tablespoons olive oil

- 2 tablespoons lemon juice

- Salt and pepper to taste

Instructions:

1. In a large bowl, combine the tuna, green beans, tomatoes, and red onion.

2. In a small bowl, whisk together the olive oil, lemon juice, salt, and pepper.

3. Pour the dressing over the tuna mixture and toss to combine.

4. Serve the tuna nicoise salad.

5. Enjoy!

Ingredients:

- 2 slices whole wheat bread

- 2 hard-boiled eggs, mashed

- 2 tablespoons mayonnaise

- 1/4 cup sliced celery

- 1/4 cup sliced green onion

- Salt and pepper to taste

Instructions:

1. Spread the mashed eggs on one slice of bread.

2. Top with the mayonnaise, celery, and green onion.

3. Season with salt and pepper.

4. Top with the other slice of bread.

5. Cut in half and serve.

6. Enjoy!

Ingredients:

- 1 whole wheat wrap

- 1/4 cup prepared falafel

- 2 tablespoons hummus

- 1/4 cup sliced cucumber

- 1/4 cup sliced tomatoes

- 1/4 cup sliced bell peppers

Instructions:

1. Preheat the oven to 350°F.

2. Place the falafel on a baking sheet and bake for 10 minutes.

3. Spread the hummus on the wrap.

4. Top with the cucumber, tomatoes, bell peppers, and baked falafel.

5. Roll the wrap up and cut in half.

6. Serve the wrap.

7. Enjoy!

4.3 HEALTHY DINNER RECIPES

[illegible]

Ingredients:

- 4 salmon fillets

- 2 tablespoons olive oil

- 2 cloves garlic, minced

- Salt and pepper, to taste

- 1 bunch asparagus, trimmed

- 1 tablespoon butter

- 1 cup cooked white rice

- 2 tablespoons chopped fresh parsley, for garnish

Instructions:

1. Preheat the grill to medium-high heat.

2. In a small bowl, combine the olive oil, garlic, salt and pepper. Brush the salmon fillets with the mixture.

3. Place the salmon and asparagus on the preheated grill, and cook for about 10 minutes, until the salmon is cooked through and the asparagus is tender.

4. Meanwhile, melt the butter in a medium saucepan over medium heat. Add the cooked rice and stir to coat.

5. Serve the grilled salmon and asparagus over the rice pilaf and garnish with fresh parsley.

Ingredients:

- 4 cod fillets

- 2 tablespoons olive oil

- 2 cloves garlic, minced

- Salt and pepper, to taste

- 2 tablespoons lemon juice

- 1 pound small potatoes, quartered

- 2 tablespoons butter

- 1 bunch broccolini, trimmed

- 2 tablespoons chopped fresh parsley, for garnish

Instructions:

1. Preheat the oven to 400°F.

2. In a small bowl, combine the olive oil, garlic, salt and pepper. Brush the cod fillets with the mixture.

3. Place the cod and potatoes on a parchment-lined baking sheet. Drizzle with the lemon juice and dot with the butter.

4. Roast in the preheated oven for 25 minutes, until the cod is cooked through and the potatoes are tender.

5. Add the broccolini to the baking sheet and roast for an additional 10 minutes.

6. Serve the cod, potatoes and broccolini and garnish with fresh parsley.

Ingredients:

- 2 tablespoons olive oil

- 1 onion, diced

- 2 cloves garlic, minced

- 2 cups cooked lentils

- 2 cups vegetable broth

- 2 carrots, diced

- 2 cups kale, chopped

- Salt and pepper, to taste

Instructions:

1. Heat the olive oil in a large saucepan over medium heat.

2. Add the onion and garlic and cook until softened, about 5 minutes.

3. Add the lentils, vegetable broth, carrots and kale. Season with salt and pepper.

4. Bring to a boil, then reduce the heat and simmer for 10 minutes, until the vegetables are tender.

5. Serve warm.

Ingredients:

- 2 tablespoons olive oil

- 2 zucchini, diced

- 2 red bell peppers, diced

- 2 cloves garlic, minced

- 1 can chickpeas, drained and rinsed

- 2 tablespoons lemon juice

- 1/4 cup chopped fresh parsley

- Salt and pepper, to taste

Instructions:

1. Preheat the oven to 400°F.

2. In a large bowl, combine the olive oil, zucchini, bell peppers and garlic. Toss to coat.

3. Arrange the vegetables on a parchment-lined baking sheet and roast for 20 minutes, until tender.

4. Add the chickpeas to the baking sheet and roast for an additional 5 minutes.

5. Transfer the roasted vegetables and chickpeas to a large bowl and add the lemon juice, parsley, salt and pepper.

6. Toss to combine and serve warm.

Ingredients:

- 2 tablespoons olive oil

- 1 eggplant, cut into 1/2-inch slices

- Salt and pepper, to taste

- 2 tomatoes, diced

- 2 tablespoons balsamic vinegar

- 2 tablespoons chopped fresh basil

Instructions:

1. Preheat the grill to medium-high heat.

2. Brush the eggplant slices with the olive oil and season with salt and pepper.

3. Place the eggplant slices on the preheated grill and cook for 5 minutes per side, until tender and lightly charred.

4. Remove the eggplant from the grill and let cool.

5. In a large bowl, combine the grilled eggplant, tomatoes, balsamic vinegar and basil.

6. Toss to combine and serve warm.

Ingredients:

- 2 tablespoons olive oil

- 1 pound boneless, skinless chicken breasts, cubed

- Salt and pepper, to taste

- 1 red onion, cut into 1-inch pieces

- 1 red bell pepper, cut into 1-inch pieces

- 1 zucchini, cut into 1-inch pieces

Instructions:

1. Preheat the grill to medium-high heat.

2. In a large bowl, combine the olive oil, chicken, salt and pepper. Toss to coat.

3. Thread the chicken and vegetables onto skewers and place on the preheated grill.

4. Grill for 10 minutes, turning occasionally, until the chicken is cooked through and the vegetables are tender.

5. Serve warm.

Ingredients:

- 2 tablespoons sesame oil

- 1 package extra-firm tofu, cubed

- 2 cloves garlic, minced

- 1 red bell pepper, sliced

- 1 carrot, sliced

- 1/2 cup snow peas

- 2 tablespoons soy sauce

- 2 tablespoons chopped fresh cilantro

Instructions:

1. Preheat the oven to 400°F.

2. In a large bowl, combine the sesame oil, tofu and garlic. Toss to coat.

3. Arrange the tofu on a parchment-lined baking sheet and bake for 20 minutes, until golden.

4. Heat a large skillet over medium heat. Add the bell pepper, carrot and snow peas and cook, stirring occasionally, until tender, about 5 minutes.

5. Add the cooked tofu and soy sauce to the skillet and cook for an additional 2 minutes.

6. Serve the stir-fry with the chopped cilantro.

Ingredients:

- 2 tablespoons olive oil

- 2 sweet potatoes, peeled and cubed

- Salt and pepper, to taste

- 2 cloves garlic, minced

- 1 cup quinoa, cooked

- 2 cups kale, chopped

- 2 tablespoons lemon juice

- 2 tablespoons chopped fresh parsley

Instructions:

1. Preheat the oven to 400°F.

2. In a large bowl, combine the olive oil, sweet potatoes, salt and pepper. Toss to coat.

3. Arrange the sweet potatoes on a parchment-lined baking sheet and roast for 25 minutes, until tender.

4. Heat a large skillet over medium heat. Add the garlic and cook until fragrant, about 1 minute.

5. Add the cooked quinoa, kale, lemon juice and sweet potatoes to the skillet and cook, stirring occasionally, until the kale is wilted, about 5 minutes.

6. Serve the quinoa with the chopped parsley.

Ingredients:

- 1 pound ground turkey

- 2 cloves garlic, minced

- 2 tablespoons chopped fresh parsley

- 2 tablespoons grated Parmesan cheese

- 1 teaspoon Italian seasoning

- Salt and pepper, to taste

- 2 cups spinach, chopped

- 2 tablespoons olive oil

Instructions:

1. Preheat the oven to 400°F.

2. In a large bowl, combine the ground turkey, garlic, parsley, Parmesan cheese, Italian seasoning, salt and pepper.

3. Mix in the spinach and form the mixture into 1-inch meatballs.

4. Place the meatballs on a parchment-lined baking sheet and drizzle with the olive oil.

5. Bake in the preheated oven for 15 minutes, until the meatballs are cooked through.

6. Serve warm.

Ingredients:

- 2 tablespoons olive oil

- 1 head cauliflower, cut into florets

- 2 teaspoons chili powder

- Salt and pepper, to taste

- 1 can chickpeas, drained and rinsed

- 2 tablespoons lemon juice

- 2 tablespoons chopped fresh parsley

Instructions:

1. Preheat the oven to 400°F.

2. In a large bowl, combine the olive oil, cauliflower, chili powder, salt and pepper. Toss to coat.

3. Arrange the cauliflower on a parchment-lined baking sheet and roast for 20 minutes, until tender.

4. Add the chickpeas to the baking sheet and roast for an additional 5 minutes.

5. Transfer the roasted cauliflower and chickpeas to a large bowl and add the lemon juice and parsley.

6. Toss to combine and serve warm.

Ingredients:

-1 ripe banana

-2 tablespoons tahini

-1 cup unsweetened almond milk

-1 teaspoon honey

Instructions:

1. Peel and slice the banana

2. Place the banana, tahini, almond milk and honey in a blender

3. Blend until smooth

Ingredients:

-2 medium zucchinis

-2 tablespoons olive oil

-1 teaspoon garlic powder

-1 teaspoon onion powder

-1 teaspoon sea salt

Instructions:

1. Preheat oven to 400°F

2. Slice the zucchinis into thin circles

3. Place the zucchini slices in a bowl and add the olive oil, garlic powder, onion powder, and salt

4. Toss to coat and spread the slices onto a baking sheet

5. Bake for 25-30 minutes, flipping halfway through

Ingredients:

-1 medium apple

-2 tablespoons peanut butter

Instructions:

1. Slice the apple into thin slices

2. Spread the peanut butter onto the slices

3. Enjoy!

Ingredients:

-1 cucumber

-1 tablespoon olive oil

-1 tablespoon lemon juice

-1 teaspoon fresh dill

-Salt and pepper to taste

Instructions:

1. Slice the cucumber into thin circles

2. In a bowl, combine the cucumber slices, olive oil, lemon juice, dill, salt, and pepper

3. Mix well and serve

Ingredients:

-1/4 cup almonds

-1/4 cup dried cranberries

-1/4 cup sunflower seeds

-1/4 cup pumpkin seeds

Instructions:

1. Place the almonds, cranberries, sunflower seeds, and pumpkin seeds in a bowl

2. Mix until combined

3. Enjoy!

Ingredients:

-1 large sweet potato

-2 tablespoons olive oil

-1 teaspoon garlic powder

-1 teaspoon onion powder

-1/2 teaspoon sea salt

Instructions:

1. Preheat oven to 425°F

2. Cut the sweet potato into thin fries

3. Place the fries in a bowl with the olive oil, garlic powder, onion powder, and salt

4. Toss to coat and spread the fries onto a baking sheet

5. Bake for 15-20 minutes, flipping halfway through

Ingredients:

-1/4 cup hummus

-1/2 cup sliced carrots

-1/2 cup sliced cucumbers

Instructions:

1. Place the hummus in a bowl

2. Add the carrots and cucumbers

3. Mix and enjoy!

Ingredients:

-2 eggs

Instructions:

1. Place the eggs in a pot and fill with cold water until the eggs are completely submerged

2. Place the pot on the stove and bring the water to a boil

3. Once the water is boiling, reduce the heat to low and simmer for 10 minutes

4. Remove the eggs from the pot and let cool

5. Enjoy!

Ingredients:

-1 cup plain Greek yogurt

-1/4 cup blueberries

-1/4 cup blackberries

Instructions:

1. Place the Greek yogurt in a bowl

2. Top with the blueberries and blackberries

3. Enjoy!

Ingredients:

-2 slices whole grain bread

-1/2 avocado

-1 teaspoon olive oil

-Salt and pepper to taste

Instructions:

1. Toast the bread

2. Mash the avocado and spread onto the toast

3. Drizzle with olive oil and season with salt and pepper

4. Enjoy!

Weekly Meal Planner

Week..............

	BREAKFAST	LUNCH	DINNER	SNACKS
MON				
TUE				
WED				
THU				
FRI				
SAT				
SUN				

Grocery List :

Weekly Meal Planner

Week...............

	BREAKFAST	LUNCH	DINNER	SNACKS
MON				
TUE				
WED				
THU				
FRI				
SAT				
SUN				

Grocery List :

Weekly Meal Planner

Week................

	BREAKFAST	LUNCH	DINNER	SNACKS
MON				
TUE				
WED				
THU				
FRI				
SAT				
SUN				

Grocery List :

Weekly Meal Planner

Week................

	BREAKFAST	LUNCH	DINNER	SNACKS
MON				
TUE				
WED				
THU				
FRI				
SAT				
SUN				

Grocery List :

Weekly Meal Planner

Week................

	BREAKFAST	LUNCH	DINNER	SNACKS
MON				
TUE				
WED				
THU				
FRI				
SAT				
SUN				

Grocery List :

Weekly Meal Planner

Week................

	BREAKFAST	LUNCH	DINNER	SNACKS
MON				
TUE				
WED				
THU				
FRI				
SAT				
SUN				

Grocery List :

Weekly Meal Planner

Week...............

	BREAKFAST	LUNCH	DINNER	SNACKS
MON				
TUE				
WED				
THU				
FRI				
SAT				
SUN				

Grocery List :
_______________ _______________ _______________
_______________ _______________ _______________
_______________ _______________ _______________
_______________ _______________ _______________
_______________ _______________ _______________
_______________ _______________ _______________

Weekly Meal Planner

Week................

	BREAKFAST	LUNCH	DINNER	SNACKS
MON				
TUE				
WED				
THU				
FRI				
SAT				
SUN				

Grocery List :

Weekly Meal Planner

Week................

	BREAKFAST	LUNCH	DINNER	SNACKS
MON				
TUE				
WED				
THU				
FRI				
SAT				
SUN				

Grocery List :

Weekly Meal Planner

Week................

	BREAKFAST	LUNCH	DINNER	SNACKS
MON				
TUE				
WED				
THU				
FRI				
SAT				
SUN				

Grocery List :
_______________   _______________   _______________
_______________   _______________   _______________
_______________   _______________   _______________
_______________   _______________   _______________
_______________   _______________   _______________
_______________   _______________   _______________

Weekly Meal Planner

Week................

	BREAKFAST	LUNCH	DINNER	SNACKS
MON				
TUE				
WED				
THU				
FRI				
SAT				
SUN				

Grocery List :

Weekly Meal Planner

Week................

	BREAKFAST	LUNCH	DINNER	SNACKS
MON				
TUE				
WED				
THU				
FRI				
SAT				
SUN				

Grocery List :
___________________ ___________________ ___________________
___________________ ___________________ ___________________
___________________ ___________________ ___________________
___________________ ___________________ ___________________
___________________ ___________________ ___________________
___________________ ___________________ ___________________

Weekly Meal Planner

Week................

	BREAKFAST	LUNCH	DINNER	SNACKS
MON				
TUE				
WED				
THU				
FRI				
SAT				
SUN				

Grocery List :

Weekly Meal Planner

Week...............

	BREAKFAST	LUNCH	DINNER	SNACKS
MON				
TUE				
WED				
THU				
FRI				
SAT				
SUN				

Grocery List :

Weekly Meal Planner

Week................

	BREAKFAST	LUNCH	DINNER	SNACKS
MON				
TUE				
WED				
THU				
FRI				
SAT				
SUN				

Grocery List :

Weekly Meal Planner

Week................

	BREAKFAST	LUNCH	DINNER	SNACKS
MON				
TUE				
WED				
THU				
FRI				
SAT				
SUN				

Grocery List :

Weekly Meal Planner

Week................

	BREAKFAST	LUNCH	DINNER	SNACKS
MON				
TUE				
WED				
THU				
FRI				
SAT				
SUN				

Grocery List :

Weekly Meal Planner

Week................

	BREAKFAST	LUNCH	DINNER	SNACKS
MON				
TUE				
WED				
THU				
FRI				
SAT				
SUN				

Grocery List :

Weekly Meal Planner

Week...............

	BREAKFAST	LUNCH	DINNER	SNACKS
MON				
TUE				
WED				
THU				
FRI				
SAT				
SUN				

Grocery List :

Weekly Meal Planner

Week................

	BREAKFAST	LUNCH	DINNER	SNACKS
MON				
TUE				
WED				
THU				
FRI				
SAT				
SUN				

Grocery List :

Weekly Meal Planner

Week.................

	BREAKFAST	LUNCH	DINNER	SNACKS
MON				
TUE				
WED				
THU				
FRI				
SAT				
SUN				

Grocery List :
_______________ _______________ _______________
_______________ _______________ _______________
_______________ _______________ _______________
_______________ _______________ _______________
_______________ _______________ _______________
_______________ _______________ _______________

Weekly Meal Planner

Week................

	BREAKFAST	LUNCH	DINNER	SNACKS
MON				
TUE				
WED				
THU				
FRI				
SAT				
SUN				

Grocery List :

Weekly Meal Planner

Week................

	BREAKFAST	LUNCH	DINNER	SNACKS
MON				
TUE				
WED				
THU				
FRI				
SAT				
SUN				

Grocery List :

Weekly Meal Planner

Week................

	BREAKFAST	LUNCH	DINNER	SNACKS
MON				
TUE				
WED				
THU				
FRI				
SAT				
SUN				

Grocery List :

Weekly Meal Planner

Week...............

	BREAKFAST	LUNCH	DINNER	SNACKS
MON				
TUE				
WED				
THU				
FRI				
SAT				
SUN				

Grocery List :

Weekly Meal Planner

Week................

	BREAKFAST	LUNCH	DINNER	SNACKS
MON				
TUE				
WED				
THU				
FRI				
SAT				
SUN				

Grocery List :

Weekly Meal Planner

Week................

	BREAKFAST	LUNCH	DINNER	SNACKS
MON				
TUE				
WED				
THU				
FRI				
SAT				
SUN				

Grocery List :

Weekly Meal Planner

Week................

	BREAKFAST	LUNCH	DINNER	SNACKS
MON				
TUE				
WED				
THU				
FRI				
SAT				
SUN				

Grocery List :

Weekly Meal Planner

Week................

	BREAKFAST	LUNCH	DINNER	SNACKS
MON				
TUE				
WED				
THU				
FRI				
SAT				
SUN				

Grocery List :

Weekly Meal Planner

Week................

	BREAKFAST	LUNCH	DINNER	SNACKS
MON				
TUE				
WED				
THU				
FRI				
SAT				
SUN				

Grocery List :

Weekly Meal Planner

Week................

	BREAKFAST	LUNCH	DINNER	SNACKS
MON				
TUE				
WED				
THU				
FRI				
SAT				
SUN				

Grocery List :

Weekly Meal Planner

Week................

	BREAKFAST	LUNCH	DINNER	SNACKS
MON				
TUE				
WED				
THU				
FRI				
SAT				
SUN				

Grocery List :

Weekly Meal Planner

Week................

	BREAKFAST	LUNCH	DINNER	SNACKS
MON				
TUE				
WED				
THU				
FRI				
SAT				
SUN				

Grocery List :

Weekly Meal Planner

Week................

	BREAKFAST	LUNCH	DINNER	SNACKS
MON				
TUE				
WED				
THU				
FRI				
SAT				
SUN				

Grocery List :

Weekly Meal Planner

Week................

	BREAKFAST	LUNCH	DINNER	SNACKS
MON				
TUE				
WED				
THU				
FRI				
SAT				
SUN				

Grocery List :

Weekly Meal Planner

Week................

	BREAKFAST	LUNCH	DINNER	SNACKS
MON				
TUE				
WED				
THU				
FRI				
SAT				
SUN				

Grocery List :

Weekly Meal Planner

Week................

	BREAKFAST	LUNCH	DINNER	SNACKS
MON				
TUE				
WED				
THU				
FRI				
SAT				
SUN				

Grocery List :

Weekly Meal Planner

Week................

	BREAKFAST	LUNCH	DINNER	SNACKS
MON				
TUE				
WED				
THU				
FRI				
SAT				
SUN				

Grocery List :

Weekly Meal Planner

Week................

	BREAKFAST	LUNCH	DINNER	SNACKS
MON				
TUE				
WED				
THU				
FRI				
SAT				
SUN				

Grocery List :

_____________ _____________ _____________
_____________ _____________ _____________
_____________ _____________ _____________
_____________ _____________ _____________
_____________ _____________ _____________
_____________ _____________ _____________

Weekly Meal Planner

Week................

	BREAKFAST	LUNCH	DINNER	SNACKS
MON				
TUE				
WED				
THU				
FRI				
SAT				
SUN				

Grocery List :

Weekly Meal Planner

Week................

	BREAKFAST	LUNCH	DINNER	SNACKS
MON				
TUE				
WED				
THU				
FRI				
SAT				
SUN				

Grocery List :

Weekly Meal Planner

Week.................

	BREAKFAST	LUNCH	DINNER	SNACKS
MON				
TUE				
WED				
THU				
FRI				
SAT				
SUN				

Grocery List :

Weekly Meal Planner

Week................

	BREAKFAST	LUNCH	DINNER	SNACKS
MON				
TUE				
WED				
THU				
FRI				
SAT				
SUN				

Grocery List :
_______________ _______________ _______________
_______________ _______________ _______________
_______________ _______________ _______________
_______________ _______________ _______________
_______________ _______________ _______________
_______________ _______________ _______________

Weekly Meal Planner

Week...............

	BREAKFAST	LUNCH	DINNER	SNACKS
MON				
TUE				
WED				
THU				
FRI				
SAT				
SUN				

Grocery List :

Weekly Meal Planner

Week................

	BREAKFAST	LUNCH	DINNER	SNACKS
MON				
TUE				
WED				
THU				
FRI				
SAT				
SUN				

Grocery List :

Weekly Meal Planner

Week................

	BREAKFAST	LUNCH	DINNER	SNACKS
MON				
TUE				
WED				
THU				
FRI				
SAT				
SUN				

Grocery List :

Weekly Meal Planner

Week................

	BREAKFAST	LUNCH	DINNER	SNACKS
MON				
TUE				
WED				
THU				
FRI				
SAT				
SUN				

Grocery List :

Weekly Meal Planner

Week................

	BREAKFAST	LUNCH	DINNER	SNACKS
MON				
TUE				
WED				
THU				
FRI				
SAT				
SUN				

Grocery List :

Weekly Meal Planner

Week...............

	BREAKFAST	LUNCH	DINNER	SNACKS
MON				
TUE				
WED				
THU				
FRI				
SAT				
SUN				

Grocery List :

Weekly Meal Planner

Week................

	BREAKFAST	LUNCH	DINNER	SNACKS
MON				
TUE				
WED				
THU				
FRI				
SAT				
SUN				

Grocery List :

Weekly Meal Planner

Week................

	BREAKFAST	LUNCH	DINNER	SNACKS
MON				
TUE				
WED				
THU				
FRI				
SAT				
SUN				

Grocery List :

Weekly Meal Planner

Week................

	BREAKFAST	LUNCH	DINNER	SNACKS
MON				
TUE				
WED				
THU				
FRI				
SAT				
SUN				

Grocery List :

www.ingramcontent.com/pod-product-compliance
Lightning Source LLC
Chambersburg PA
CBHW050825260726
48660CB00004B/1616